T0167053

A FOOD JUNKIE'S
Guide to Recovery

A FOOD JUNKIE'S
Guide to Recovery

Lisa Parks Silks

iUniverse LLC
Bloomington

A FOOD JUNKIE'S GUIDE TO RECOVERY
OVERCOMING A LIFETIME OF EMOTIONAL EATING

iUniverse books may be ordered through booksellers or by contacting:

iUniverse
1663 Liberty Drive
Bloomington, IN 47403
www.iuniverse.com
1-800-Authors (1-800-288-4677)

Because of the dynamic nature of the Internet, any web addresses or links contained in this book may have changed since publication and may no longer be valid. The views expressed in this work are solely those of the author and do not necessarily reflect the views of the publisher, and the publisher hereby disclaims any responsibility for them.

ISBN: 978-1-4917-0621-3 (sc)
ISBN: 978-1-4917-0623-7 (hc)
ISBN: 978-1-4917-0622-0 (e)

Library of Congress Control Number: 2013915968

Printed in the United States of America.

iUniverse rev. date: 9/18/2013

*This book is dedicated to my daughter,
Jess, the love of my life.*

Contents

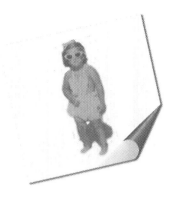

Acknowledgments

My love and gratitude to those who made this book possible, whether they know it or not:

God, my savior and constant companion. My heart overflows with gratitude.

Jessica Silks, my daughter, for smart advice and invaluable support and for always loving me "to peisus."

Linda Adams, my sister and best friend, for encouraging me to go deeper. I couldn't have done this without you, Lin!

Frances Lombardo, my aunt and godmother, for a lifetime of loving care.

Sister Joan Reilly, my counselor and friend, for the most precious conversations of my life.

Debbie Locke, a dear family friend, the angel who led me back to Sister Joan.

Anne Nickerson, my treasured friend, for sage advice and wholehearted encouragement.

Dr. Angelee Carta, my physician, for her generosity and loving care when I was unemployed, uninsured, and deeply depressed.

Dr. Jeffrey L. Cohen, my former work partner, for his integrity and generosity.

Joyce Rupp, writer and speaker, for poetry that speaks the language of my soul.

Ellen DeGeneres, talk show host/comic/author/spreader of joy and good cheer, for making me laugh and dance when times were really hard.

Joel Osteen, author and pastor of Lakewood Church in Texas, for books that lifted me up when I was down and out. Your words continue to inspire and strengthen my faith every day.

Oprah Winfrey, media royalty and philanthropist, for lighting the way for others with her own spiritual evolution.

Neighbors on my walking routes who offer a friendly greeting, especially Kristy Stone at the far end of my full route, for her friendship and encouragement.

The morning crews at my favorite haunts while I was writing:

The Cosmic Omelet (Manchester, CT), especially Tiffany and Justin, for treating me like a VIP.
Mitchell's Restaurant (Vernon, CT), especially Kate and Tori, for making me feel like family.
Shady Glen (Parkade-Manchester, CT), especially Lana, for her kindness and encouragement.

The iUniverse team, for their expertise, exceptional responsiveness, and friendliness.

My entire family, living and passed, for loving me at any and every size.

BEFORE

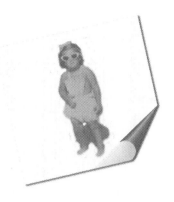

The Earliest Years

In the small cupboard over the refrigerator, I discovered two boxes of candy tucked behind a sack of flour. My little eyes widened as I saw that each box held at least fifty cubed pieces, each about the size of my thumbnail, individually wrapped in clear cellophane. Some looked like dark chocolate, some like caramel.

I jumped down off the kitchen chair and stepped over to the window above the sink. I pulled back the curtain and peered out like a spy in a "007" movie, as if an enemy secret agent might be hiding in the lilac bushes. Assured that there were no cars in the driveway—and thus no grown-ups in the house—I climbed back up on the chair and nabbed two pieces of candy, which I stuck in my pocket, along with a tag from the candy maker. After carefully replacing the chair under the kitchen table in precisely its original position, I skulked to my room like a criminal.

Even though I was certain no one else was home, I closed and locked my bedroom door before pulling the treats from my pocket. Making as little noise as possible, I meticulously peeled away the cellophane from the first morsel and popped it into my mouth. It was indeed caramel-flavored, with a consistency similar to fudge, and quite yummy. After quickly downing the first, I did the same with the darker chocolate, this time noticing an odd aftertaste beginning to bubble up in my saliva. As I ate, I read the tag: "These chewable dietary supplements are intended to suppress the appetite when eaten thirty minutes prior to each meal." Oh, jeez! These were for my mother's latest diet!

They were surprisingly tasty for diet food. Just like the real thing, except for that aftertaste. As far as I could tell, they didn't affect my appetite one bit. I stole two more the next day, and the day after that, and the day after that. With so many spilling out of each box, I doubted my mother would notice a few missing. If she did, she never let on. I don't remember whether I confessed, but I doubt it.

♥

I was about eight years old when I ate those diet supplements like candy. I'm fifty-six now and have only just begun to understand my relationship with food.

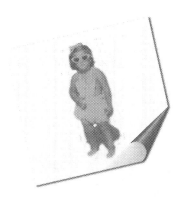

Introduction

Hi, my name is Lisa, and I am an addict. Food is my drug of choice, the substance with which I self-medicate. Mine is an emotional addiction that has plagued me since I was a child. If my relationship with food were a scripted drama, it would be easy to act out. With every emotional scene, the parenthetical stage direction would look like this: [*Stuffs face with food*].

Character is stressed … she eats. [*Stuffs face with food*]
Character is sad … she eats. [*Stuffs face with food*]
Character is angry … she eats. [*Stuffs face with food*]
Character is {every other emotion possible} … she eats …
You get the picture.

The specific foods I use to salve my wounds may change from scene to scene, but the fact remains: I eat my feelings. This unhealthy way of coping has led to years upon years of emotional eating and, ultimately, a food addiction.

I will likely open myself up to criticism for speaking of food addiction as fact. It is a controversial, highly complex topic that seems only recently to have drawn enough attention to compel the research needed to support or disprove it. Though the jury is a long way from a verdict, there are many, like me, who believe that some brains are wired for food addiction. While healthy people consciously overindulge once in a while, a food addict does so incessantly, without deliberate thought. It's hard to resist our cravings, and harder still to stop eating foods we love. Research may someday prove that certain foods raise levels of dopamine ("the pleasure chemical") in some brains to excess, creating intense feelings of pleasure associated with those foods, motivating continued eating—even when one is full. We yearn to re-create the feelings of pleasure that food has provided. That's the crux of the problem.

This book represents my opinions only, based on what I've read, interviews I've heard, and an examination of my behaviors over fifty-plus years. The truth is, at this point it doesn't matter a fig to me whether or not food addiction is a proven scientific condition. I'm not one to get caught up in science or semantics. I'm just a regular person who has battled obesity throughout my adulthood, trying my best to understand why I eat compulsively. And more important, trying to change that behavior.

♥

If I had to guess, I'd say I have been on at least one diet every year for a good thirty years. All told, I'm sure I've lost and regained at least 250 pounds. Staggering!

When I first started tackling my addiction a year ago, I weighed 230 pounds and wore a size 22. For a 5'4" frame, 230 is a scary number. There are contestants on *The Biggest Loser* who start with a number like that and look just like I did, with blobs of fat spilling out over bra straps and waistbands and a huge belly making breathing and movement difficult. Medical experts say that weight around our midsection is the most dangerous weight to carry because of the strain it puts on the heart. As someone who is not a medical expert, I can tell you it *feels* extremely uncomfortable. Unless you are lying down, there is always a big, unwelcome obstruction sitting right in the middle of your body that makes it hard—even impossible at times—to lean over, squat, sit, or cross your legs with any kind of finesse.

Like the gum-chomping Violet Beauregard in Willy Wonka's candy factory, I often felt like a pair of floundering arms and legs protruding from a big, round, plump, blueberry body, rolling around out of control. In the movie, Wonka calmly tells Violet's father, "She has to be squeezed immediately before she explodes." If only it were that easy! I was headed for serious trouble if I continued to carry that kind of weight.

As I write this, I weigh 173 pounds and wear a size 14, and there's no turning back. Since you are reading this, you may have a weight problem too or care about someone who does. Maybe you have been through a few diet ordeals yourself. Perhaps you are also an addict who has felt as helpless and discouraged as I have through the years. If so, I feel your pain, believe me. I hope my experience will help you.

There were many times throughout my life when I blamed my mother for my food issues, pointing to her dysfunctional relationship with food and saying, "See—no wonder I have this problem." Unfortunately, she dealt with the same addiction and struggle I have faced for years. Unwittingly, she passed the torch to me. But ultimately I chose to carry the torch. I'm no psychiatrist, but my experience and the collective experience of my obese sisterhood tells me that, somewhere along the line, my mother—like me and maybe like you—discovered that some problems are easier to feed than to solve. If you stuff it down, it can't be seen and thus can be more easily ignored and avoided.

The truth is, we can blame anything and anybody, even *every*thing and *every*body, until we're blue in the face—and plump as a Wonka berry, as it were! But it's in our true best interest to instead do some fervent soul-searching about the overeater within. That's where the truth resides. Facing and understanding that truth has proven just as important to sustained weight loss as diet and exercise—maybe even more so.

Naturally, I looked to my childhood first. Not to place blame, but to learn about the roots of my relationship with food. I'm guessing what I saw there will resonate with you. In deepest reflection, I came face-to-face with my inner food junkie. We have journeyed arm in arm ever since. Through our new alliance, we have uncovered some significant details that have led to a new life lived in unity and peace. Together, we have discovered our path to "clean" living. Without her, I could not have found it.

I hope my story will encourage others to seek out and befriend their inner junkie, stop feeling bad about themselves and their tendencies to overeat, develop a healthier relationship with food over time, and kick their habitual emotional responses to food. My experience has done that for me and has vastly improved my overall health and well-being. That's what I hope it will do for you too.

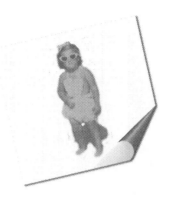

Glimpses of Childhood:
MEETING MY INNER JUNKIE

In my childhood home on Cole Street, a crawl space connected the two upstairs bedrooms. On one side was the room I shared with my big sister; on the other was my brother's room, which became mine several years later when he left for college. To a five-year-old, the crawl space was a long, dark tunnel of cobwebs, where ghouls and goblins hovered, shifting incessantly from one doorway to the other throughout the night, primed for entry, raring to frighten little girls. Much to my amazement, just a couple of short years later, I bravely smushed the cobwebs with a wet paper towel and took rights of ownership with very little fear. Now it was my long, dark tunnel of stillness and secrecy.

In that quiet little space, I set up camp, stocking it with pillows and blankets and puzzles and coloring books and doodads worthy of hours of undetected solitary play. I wrote poems and made up jokes for my stuffed animals' amusement. It seems I may have interacted with an invisible playmate, but I recognize her now as my inner junkie.

During the late-afternoon hours between school and dinner, we crept in and out of our tiny clubhouse every so often, as the stale air required. I had to scootch out carefully so as not to hit my head on the slanted ceiling where the eaves came together with the wall. I made clandestine trips to the kitchen for snacks. We pigged out on stacks of graham crackers smeared with soft, sweet butter and creamy peanut butter, served on a china saucer with a fancy silver knife. In retrospect, that seems astonishingly grown-up and civilized for a seven-year-old. Perhaps I thought it gave my little tunnel an elegant refinement, making the act of sneaking snacks seem less egregious.

Weeks of covert operations later, my mother discovered my hideout in a most distressing manner. My snacks had drawn ants. Thankfully, I was not there at the time she traced them to my private oasis, where she found a streaming parade of those industrious little critters crawling on and around her china and silver pieces. To this day, I'm not sure whether I was reprimanded for hiding, snacking, or using the good china. I suspect it was mostly about the ants, but to my busted little heart it was a trifecta of offenses for which I carried heaps of guilt for days.

♥

My parents both worked full-time. In those days, there were few working mothers; all the mothers within at least a ten-block radius (your whole world as a child) were stay-at-home moms. In fact, the term "stay-at-home mom" didn't exist yet, since working mothers were the exception. When she wasn't sick, my mom was a brilliant whirling dervish of energy who wanted the finer things in life for her family of five. My parents' teacher's salaries didn't make us rich, by any means. But we wanted for little and had a lot of things many other families did not.

One of our luxury items was a storage freezer. It was the size and shape of a refrigerator, but it sat horizontally, and everything in it was rock hard. When you opened the lid, a rush of frozen air swirled around like puffs of clouds above the food. Sometimes you'd have to fan the mist away before you could determine what was inside. My parents were thrilled at the money they saved by buying and storing large quantities of meat bought in bulk directly from the butcher. He supplied a drawing of a cow and a pig, with arrows charting all the different edible sections by name, and my parents would put in their quarter-year order accordingly. It likely paid for itself in pork chops in no time.

The freezer was stored on the enclosed porch that extended across the back of our house. It was easy to get foods in and out of it, making it convenient for both daily use and long-term storage. After holidays, any leftover cookies and pastries were tightly wrapped in double layers of tin foil and hidden among the steaks and hamburgers. There were sometimes Christmas cookies to be found there, the procurement of which became a game of espionage. I had to devise reasons for going out onto the porch without raising suspicion. To avoid being seen, timing was critical. My inner junkie was exceptionally good at these games.

I snuck the cookies out two by two and ate them frozen. They were divine, even icy cold and stiffly solid. After seconds in my mouth, they'd soften up beautifully and provide lasting, chewy, delicious satisfaction. Unfortunately, I was reckless with the rewrapping. Kids don't have much patience for that. It didn't take long for my mother to realize that I was delving into the goodies. She was not happy about it. "Those are for *special occasions!*" she cried, looking at me wide-eyed, like I'd committed a mortal sin and stood in the very clutches of Satan himself. Whew! The drama.

I apologized profusely and slunk away. I was sincerely sorry for upsetting my mom, but I had a hard time feeling sorry that I had eaten the cookies. They were so delicious that I was pretty sure it was worth whatever punishment might follow. As it turned out, I received no punishment, and knowing it would be forgotten within a few weeks, my inner junkie had already begun plotting our next strategy for acquisition.

♥

Since my folks were teachers, our summers were extraordinary. We took road trips in our Country Squire station wagon, even traveling across the entire country one summer with another of our luxury items in tow: a pop-up Nimrod camping trailer. We visited faraway relatives and saw all the wonders of America.

I was only six years old, so one of the few wonders I remember without prompting is being allowed by relatives in Texas to have all the watermelon I could eat, enjoyed in big, full quarters, one after the other, seed-spitting optional. Fun! I had so much watermelon, I wet their bed that night. That kind of humiliation keeps a memory alive.

Whether camping or close to home, we spent countless hours on the beach. Saltwater virtually runs in my veins. As the story goes, we started out camping in the back of a one-room ice house near the Connecticut shore. I have no recollection of that. Some years later, we rented the upstairs of a three-bedroom duplex for a whole summer month, right on the water at Middle Beach in Westbrook. Years later, we shifted to Misquamicut Beach in Westerly, Rhode Island, extending our stay to six weeks and eventually buying a cottage of our own, where we spent full summers of bliss!

The Ortisi-LaBella family owned the big property in Westbrook. They lived in a house behind the duplex for the entire summer. A small, primly gardened courtyard sat between the houses, where we all often came together after the day's adventures. Tory was my best friend. He was the grandson of Mama and Papa Ortisi. We spent all our daytime hours together swimming; dodging jellyfish; bailing water from a decrepit, leaky rowboat; combing the beach for unique shells and rocks; and dangling mussels on a string-laced stick to catch crabs off the rock jetty. At night, we ate s'mores or made Jiffy Pop popcorn. We played cards and had dance-offs. We laughed ourselves nearly to death. When we were called inside, we rushed through our nightly rituals, threw on our pajamas, and skipped off to our bedroom windows across the courtyard from one another, where we continued our chatter long distance through Dixie cups on a string until we heard Papa shouting, "Zitto! Sleep, sleep!"

The yard was always filled with sweet aromas from Mama Ortisi's kitchen. She was a first-generation Italian who spoke very little English; her language was food. And boy oh boy, could she talk! Surprisingly, her grandson was as thin as a blade of grass. But then, he was always in a tizzy, buzzing about here and there, doing this and that. He never stood still, that one. So even though we ate like there was no tomorrow, he stayed rail thin, while my inner junkie got fat and happy.

To this day, the smell of sweet Italian peppers frying in olive oil still causes an undeniable pool of drool to collect in my mouth. Pepper-and-egg grinders, handmade ricotta ravioli, eggplant cooked to perfection and layered with fresh mozzarella ... everything made fresh with herbs from the garden and the cook's boundless love, served up like a romance novel.

♥

My mother was also an excellent cook. Her Italian meals rivaled Mama Ortisi's. When she cooked, her Naples roots proved unbreakable, and she channeled all the women of her heritage who had taught her the language of food.

Religious holidays were grand feasts. My large, extended family came together and gorged on massive quantities of food: antipasto piled high with pepperoni, provolone, genoa salami, and other assorted meats and cheeses; a vast array of olives, dates, nuts, fruits, and crudités; caprese salad with fresh mozzarella, ripe tomato slices, and fresh basil leaves; and, of course, a variety of child-friendly chips and dips. Torrone nougat candy and shiny, colorful ribbon candy were artfully set out in fancy glassware, strategically placed in all the high-traffic areas around the house. Dinner was comprised of lasagna, piled high; seemingly endless quantities of sausage and meatballs; and freshly baked, oven-toasted garlic bread. There was salad and broccoli—other stuff too—but they had no appeal whatsoever until I was much older.

The desserts came from an authentic Italian bakery on Franklin Avenue in Hartford: cannoli, cookies, spumoni, rum cake. I may have heard more Italian spoken there than any time at the Ortisis'. Believe it or not, I didn't eat a cannoli until I was in my twenties. I couldn't imagine why people would eat dry pastry filled with cold cheese when they could be eating divinely sweet cookies!

Food Junkie's Aside: Gooey, chewy macaroon-style, made with almond paste, sprinkled with pine nuts or colored red and green and topped with a maraschino cherry. Oh my!

When I finally tried a cannoli, I chided myself for what I'd been missing all those years. I'd had no idea they were sweetened!

The people at the grown-ups' table had mounds of cookies and bakery boxes full of pastries and could eat all they wanted without scrutiny. The kids' table got one small, dessert-plate-sized allotment of cookies to share, and the few times we were allowed to eat cannolis, they were cut in half and assigned one section to a customer. Only now do I realize I probably could have traded my share for an extra cookie. All those years, I just gave it away to the cousin who asked most sweetly. Dang! I couldn't wait till the day I would be allowed at the grown-ups' table.

♥

I was exposed to a lot of fun activities as a child, especially during the more carefree summers, but it's the food I remember enjoying most. One special trip we took periodically over the years was to Old Sturbridge Village, one of the country's oldest and largest living history museums. It brought to life early New England from 1790–1840. We could watch the making of teapots and lanterns in the tin shop, see apples pressed into cider by horsepower in the mill, and explore buildings and homes with historians in costume. We watched sheep being sheared and marveled at the sight of their wool being spun and dyed. The blacksmith forged new shoes for the horses. Butter was freshly churned. Bread, pies, and cookies baked in the flames of firelight in a dark, dirt-floored kitchen, with samples available for tasting. It was a world of exciting exhibits and fascinating activities!

With all that I would see and experience, what I looked forward to most about our Sturbridge trips was the stop on the way home at Hebert's Candy Shop. Hebert's was in a big, stone castle laid out with a gigantic assortment of freshly made chocolates, vast varieties of fudge, and seasonal treats.

In keeping with the Sturbridge theme, they made chocolate lollipops in animal shapes like the lambs we had just seen at the farm. I loved peering through the glass cases at all the scrumptious goodies. Knowing I could select just one treat necessitated long moments of contemplation. I paused admiringly over the nonpareils, peanut butter taffy kisses, and rich, milk-chocolate-covered, malted milk balls but always ended up delightedly choosing velvety, rich white chocolate on a stick. So exotic!

♥

No one would claim I was a finicky eater in general, but my Auntie Fran and Uncle Joe learned well the few foods I couldn't stomach. When my mother was ill, which was often, especially in my earliest years of life, I stayed overnight at their house. My little cousin Richard was like a living doll, adorably cute and sweet, and we had a lot of fun together. I'm sure I was traumatized by having to be away from my mother so often at such a young age, but I felt loved there, all the same.

One of my strongest memories of those overnight visits is of Uncle Joe's soft-boiled eggs served in little, individual, white and red porcelain egg cups. I've never known anyone else ever who had egg cups in their kitchenware, but I'm pretty sure they saw considerable use at Uncle Joe's. I *loathed* soft-boiled eggs! We sat down at the table together for breakfast, which was quite special and lovely, giving my broken, interrupted life the illusion of an *Ozzie and Harriet* episode. The egg cups were stylishly served on a woven place mat, with spoon and cloth napkin neatly tucked beside it, accompanied by a small plate of perfectly toasted bread with just a hint of butter and orange marmalade. Uncle Joe slurped his egg up with delight; clearly, this was a house specialty he made for the occasion. To this, my reaction was "Eeeewwww! Do I have to eat that?"

The answer was an unequivocal "Yes!" In fact, I would not be allowed to leave the table until I had eaten my egg. This was a shock—at home, I'd never been required to eat anything I didn't like. Encouraged, yes, but required—never. Here with my aunt and uncle, I was expected to become an honored member of the "clean-plate club" who at all times eats the foods she or he is served, even the disgusting, nutritious ones. They tried desperately to impress upon me that this was good for me and important for a healthy, growing body. Oh Lord, I gag even now at the thought of that runny, slimy-looking cup full of yuck!

At some point in the standoff, my aunt acquiesced, much to my uncle's chagrin. Maybe she felt I was already suffering enough as a castaway with a sick mother. I was convinced I would throw up right there at the table if I tried to eat the egg, so I believed I was actually doing everyone a huge favor by staunchly refusing.

Another source of controversy was spinach. They probably got Richard to eat his by convincing him he would grow up big and strong like Popeye, the spinach-loving sailor man. That would likely appeal to a young boy, but I was a girl with no desire to smoke a pipe or have tattooed forearms the size of tree trunks. I found the very smell of cooked spinach horrendous! I couldn't possibly put that foul aroma right under my nose and into my mouth! My wriggling torso and contorted facial expressions said it all. If this was the classic stuff of nutritious and good-for-you foods, I'd be having none of it, thank you. I'd rather be pudgy Winnie-the-Pooh savoring gooey honey and all things sweet!

I adored my aunt and uncle and would return to them many years later for sanctuary when I hit bottom following a short, tumultuous marriage. I appeared unannounced one day at their doorstep with a two-year-old daughter, a seven-year-old cat, and a rusting, beat-up Oldsmobile stuffed with all my earthly possessions. They took me in and lovingly cared for me just as they always had.

Food was at the heart of everything. Every disappointment; every celebration; every event, good or bad, was highlighted by what we ate. A successful dance recital, a good report card, helping with chores and the like, meant pizza from Vic's, ice cream sundaes at Friendly's, or maybe fresh éclairs from the Parkade bakery. A lost part in the school play or a misunderstanding with a good friend might result in my then-favorite dinner of spaghetti with butter and parmesan cheese, beef stew with dumplings, or the rare treat of homemade French fries.

Even my glorious days at the beach conjure images of special sweets. As far as the beach itself was concerned, I could likely tell you more about the thrill of hearing the bells of the Italian lemon ice truck as it made its way around the neighborhood; or about the saltwater taffy you could only get at the shore, where you could watch it being twisted and stretched in the storefront window; or the penny candy store in the center of town, where you could always beg a few coins from your parents for Squirrel Nut Zippers and Mary Janes. I could pop sweets in my mouth until I was sick to my stomach without thinking twice, never once giving a thought to any *feelings* behind it. I certainly never thought of food as healing, but without question it had great power to do so.

I only remember my mother having heart issues once during our stays at the beach. I was usually sheltered from these events. Thankfully, this was not a week my dad had stayed back in Manchester to tutor kids in math or sell *World Book Encyclopedias* for extra money. He didn't let me go upstairs to see my mother, but I was witness to the chaos around us and had never seen my father's complexion so gray. I felt alarmed to my bones—and invisible. Someone in the main house called 911, and Tory's mom, Sara, shooed me and Tory to the street to watch for the ambulance and direct it into the driveway.

I stood by as the medics carried my mom down the outside stairs from the second floor, tightly bound on a stretcher. It was tenuous and scary. I don't remember whether she was conscious or whether either of us spoke. The world had stopped on its axis, and everything went into slow motion like a *Twilight Zone* montage.

I felt a tremendous weight on my chest and worked incredibly hard to hold back tears and the sudden hysteria I was feeling inside. I started a fight with Tory, throwing lots of antagonistic words at him, none of which I meant, while the ambulance drove my mom and dad away into the distance. My misdirected rage confused Tory, but he remained loving and kind. He refused to fight back.

Mama Ortisi cooked up a storm that afternoon. Every chance she got, she drew me into her kitchen for "a bite" to eat. She clutched me in her arms, holding me close, almost suffocating me in her oversized bosoms, ranting tearfully in Italian. Sara ordered people to get me "a little something" every ten minutes, all day and night. "Go, Pa, a little ice cream will cheer her up!" "Salvatore, bring our Lisa a little plate of pasta—she'll feel better." God bless them. They had no idea they were force-feeding a junkie.

There's a reason we label certain childhood foods as "comfort food." Simply and obviously, it's where many of us turn for just that—comfort. Clearly, food is an integral part of my childhood memories, so it makes sense that food is where I turn for emotional balance, especially when feeling something unpleasant. Fear, disappointment, anger, illness … all good reasons to overeat, according to my twisted way of thinking—or of *not* thinking, I should say.

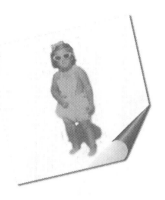

Emotional Eating

Emotional eaters are driven to stuff delicious foods into their mouths with reckless abandon. As a child, food was a familiar friend when I was lonely, a source of pleasure when there was pain. Emotional eating became the habit of a lifetime for me, the yin and yang, a joy and a curse. The taste and the pleasure response in the brain provided the joy. The curse would come later, when I came to my senses and felt shame and guilt at my excesses and increasing waistline. To cast off those destructive feelings, I'd (over)eat again, in an unconscious effort to replace them with more pleasurable feelings. A vicious cycle, to say the least.

When we're eating our emotions, we generally don't even realize we're eating at all. We get so wrapped up in the tasty sensations and the positive feelings stimulated by food, we just start feeling good again. It's that feel-good stimulation in our brains that creates and feeds the addiction.

A great deal of mindless eating goes on in a food junkie's life. By the time I was an adult, I had become an expert at mindless eating, especially when work was stressful, which was most of the time. I'd keep a large jar of Hershey's kisses or jelly beans or some other quick-to-pop-in-the-mouth sweet on my desk, and by the end of the day I would be surprised to find the container completely empty. Of course, colleagues enjoyed a few once in a while, but usually I'd have finished them all off on my own without thinking. I didn't even notice that I was eating them.

I would also do a lot of mindless eating right after work, usually starting the minute I got home, though sometimes a drive-through would draw me in for a good, quick, salty French-fry fix first. This was especially true when I'd been barraged by conflict at work or when the commute home had been particularly long and aggressive. Before supper was made, I'd already have eaten nearly a full meal of calories just in nibbling and snacking. I never even thought about it. And it didn't stop me from eating my dinner as well.

When I got clean and eliminated mindless eating from my day, it made a sizable difference in my calorie consumption and contributed to my weight-loss success. Over the next few days, try to be conscious of everything you put in your mouth. You might be amazed at the number of mindless calories you're eating. Unfortunately, even if they go down like fiction, they show up on our bodies as fact.

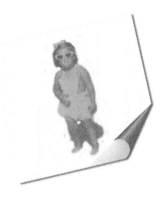

Misophonia

Here's another significant reality that goaded my inner junkie:

Eating created all manner of sounds that got on my mother's nerves like nails on a chalkboard, so "Chew with your mouth closed" was a principal commandment in our house. It was reiterated a gazillion times. Crunching, chomping, slurping, and lip-smacking were all dire transgressions that would result in stern reminders to watch our manners.

Gum-snapping was outright scandalous! My mother was driven so insane by that sound, she tried to shame people who chewed gum in her presence out of ever doing it again by telling them how ridiculous it made them look—"like cows chewing their cud." She'd not have it—definitely not in her classroom and certainly not in her home.

There's a name for this now. It's called misophonia. It occurs when a common, repetitive noise, like chewing, water dripping, or someone drumming their fingers, causes even the most level-headed and kind-hearted people to be driven up the wall. Unfortunately, I developed misophonia too, likely due to the severity of my mother's condition. To varying degrees, sufferers are said to experience "an eruption of emotions associated with these sounds." We do everything we can to stop or avoid them.

This was a Vesuvius-sized revelation during my recovery! My mother's misophonia had had a tremendous impact on the formation of my inner junkie, who, as junkies do, encouraged me to act in secrecy. I gladly went along to avert the chances of a chastising look or a scolding. Imagine the effect on a child if every time she eats, she is told to be quiet. Wow!

I've come to terms with this without harboring anger or resentment toward my mom. Forgiveness of self and others is a key step in a junkie's recovery. We all do the best we can. If you need help with forgiveness, I recommend a pastoral counselor. Mine did wonders for me.

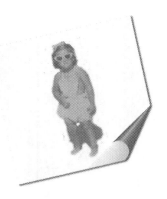

The Long and Winding Road:
WEIGHT-LOSS PROGRAMS

The truth is, a lot of weight-loss programs work. I've pretty much done them all, and I've had success on most of them.

As an avid meat eater and cheese lover, I liked the Atkins Diet. By drastically restricting carbohydrates, you go into a state of ketosis, which changes your body from a carbohydrate-burning machine to a fat-burning machine. While getting into ketosis, I could eat all the meat and cheese I wanted during the first weeks of the program, which was heaven. I was never hungry, and if I wanted, I could just eat cheese smothered in cheese. Nirvana!

> **Food Junkie's Aside:** There's a restaurant in my hometown called Shady Glen that is famous for its cheeseburgers. There's also grilled cheese right on the menu. They throw three or four slices on a hot, greasy griddle, and as the cheese melts, they curl the corners and bend it into these delectable works of art with just the right blend of gooey and crunchy. Genius!

Anyway ... I did very well on Atkins and could always lose weight in the early stages of the program. It's when I started putting other foods back in my diet that I would struggle with control and making choices and would eventually put all the weight back on. Believe it or not, I lowered my cholesterol on Atkins, and I think it's a great plan if you do it the way you're supposed to and can sustain it.

I was successful with Weight Watcher's too. I have followed that program nearly a dozen times in my life and lost a noteworthy amount of weight each time. But I always grew tired of the weigh-ins and meetings, which seemed after a while like the same dialogue over and over again. Plus, as long as I counted the "points" for it, I could eat anything

I wanted, so I did. That often resulted in my eating an unbalanced menu of food each day, and I seemed to be hungry all the time. So I quit that too and put all the weight back on, plus more, every time. I went back to the program repeatedly, which is a testament to its effectiveness. It's one of the best weight-loss programs I know of, and I wish all my WW sisters and brothers great success! It just wasn't the final answer for me.

Optifast was an intense experience. This was a hospital-monitored liquid diet consisting of months of ingesting nothing but shakes of powder mixed with water or diet soda. Egads! When I think about it now, that was just destined to fail! Surprisingly, for me a liquid diet was actually easier than it sounds, because there were no food choices to be made. Zero. I couldn't overeat or eat the "wrong" foods; there was simply *no food allowed*! That was the first time I ever lost enough to reach my "goal weight." I developed a kidney stone in the process, and as regular solid food was reintroduced, I eventually gained all the weight back. So goal, schmoal. It wasn't worth it.

Those are just three diet programs that I've tried. There have been countless others along the way. Like I said, I've dieted over and over again for more years than I care to think about. At the start of a new year, on my birthday, or with the arrival of spring (in anticipation of showing more skin), I started another diet, always starting on a Monday and usually bingeing over the prior weekend to get in a last blast of Chinese food or whatever else I feared being unable to eat again. I'd typically scarf down two or three pints of Ben & Jerry's ice cream the Saturday and Sunday before each diet.

> *Food Junkie's Aside: Cherry Garcia, with big, luscious black cherries and massive chunks of rich dark chocolate. Delectable!*

If you're keeping track, you know three of the great loves of my life: chewy sweets, cheese, and ice cream, also known as triggers for ridiculous overconsumption! If you're wondering why I have allowed my inner junkie to chime in with those little tidbits of thought, let me explain. First, it's almost impossible to quiet her when speaking of certain foods. Second, it's important to understand that my passion for food has not been repressed. I still love feel-good foods, and I still *eat* feel-good foods, but it's become a whispered aside rather than a thunderous bellow.

Around the time of my fifty-fifth birthday, everything changed. I found another missing link in all my prior attempts at weight management. I started living consciously moment to moment, which led to eating meal-by-meal, losing weight pound-by-pound, and walking step-by-step to a whole new life.

♥

There are components to my journey beyond food that I believe will help others, whether they are food addicts or not, but understand that I was focused on my own compulsion toward emotional eating. That's what I have overcome. And weight loss was a critical task before me. So that's where I began.

Perhaps this is a good time to talk a little about the physical mechanics of my recovery ...

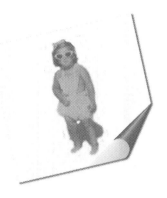

You and Your Body

Again, please understand that I'm not an expert in the field of nutrition. I'm not a physician, nor do I have any clinical knowledge on which you should rely. There are fabulous sources of information in local libraries and bookstores and on the Internet. I use webmd.com and ask.com often when doing research or estimating nutritional information. There are countless resources on the Internet. I don't endorse any particular material or any one site. You should use your best judgment to decide what's right for you.

Your doctor would be an excellent resource, since you both have an intimate knowledge of your particular health conditions. I have hypothyroidism and had high cholesterol at the time I started my new life; you may have diabetes or blood-pressure issues or other physical conditions that would dictate what is best for your body in terms of your intake of calories, sugar, sodium, cholesterol, etc.

But before we even talk about food, here are a few mind-altering essentials to my recovery.

DURING

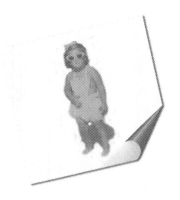

The Essentials:
THROW THESE DIET MISTAKES
OUT THE WINDOW

I mean it. If you're interested in weight loss, *throw these diet mistakes out the window!*

Mistake #1: The End Goal

Every time I have dieted, the very first step has been setting a weight-loss goal. In some programs, they write it down so you can look at it every now and again to remind yourself of where you want to be. That seems like a reasonable beginning; if you were taking a trip, you'd certainly want to know your final destination. But I've come to understand that that was the first mistake in all my weight-loss efforts.

In the past thirty years or so, I've had at least fifty pounds to lose at any given time—often seventy-five or more. That's *daunting*! So anytime I set a long-term end goal, I was pretty overwhelmed from the get-go. Facing a big weight-loss number like that, I was discouraged before I even began. During recovery, I threw big weight targets out the window. Naturally, I know where I want to end up, but the only goal I am striving for at any given time is to lose a pound. One pound. When that pound is lost, I set out to lose another. One pound at a time, never looking any further ahead.

A pound is doable, right? Right! Anybody can lose *one pound*. I'm guessing that, like me, you've proven that for yourself time and time again. So at any given moment, instead of feeling overwhelmed by the enormity of, say, a sixty-pound weight-loss goal, I was set up for success, pound by single pound.

Recovery Words to Live By

Decide on your ultimate destination; then deliberately and enthusiastically embrace every step of the journey. Celebrate every single pound you lose!

Mistake #2: The Timetable

With fifty or sixty or seventy-five plus-pounds to lose, I had to face the fact that, unless I wanted to go to formidable extremes with diet and exercise, weight loss of that magnitude would realistically take at least a year, possibly two. That's also daunting! Could I work that hard and deprive myself for that long? The thought of dieting (translation: restriction and sacrifice) for a whole year or more was positively demoralizing! So again, I'd practically give up before I even got started.

Do you know what that timetable would cause me to do? I'd continuously calculate dubious weight losses in my head. The running monologue would say, "If I can lose 'x' pounds in 'x' days, I will weigh 'x' by 'such-and-such a date.'" By thinking this way, always looking a ways down the road, I missed important steps in the journey and caused myself needless pressure and the repeated disappointment of not meeting unrealistic expectations. When "such-and-such date" came around, if I hadn't lost "x," which more than likely I would not have, I'd feel like a failure. After a few failures, I'd stop looking at any short-term success I may have had, proclaim the diet ineffective and the effort futile, and I'd quit.

During recovery, I threw timetables out the window. If it took me a day, a week, or a month to lose that pound, by God I was going to embrace that one-pound loss! I just wanted to lose a pound, period. Whatever number was on the scale one morning created my goal for the next morning ... and the morning after that … and the morning after that, which was simply to be one pound lighter.

As soon as I was one pound lighter, whenever that happened, I'd feel fantastic. Mission accomplished! Excitedly, I'd set my new goal to be one pound lighter than that. When I stopped setting impractical, idealistic timetables, losing weight seemed easier, and most important, I was successfully meeting my goal much faster than I would have if the goal were ten pounds or more. Why celebrate one ten when you can celebrate ten ones? I was a success story with every new pound, and it felt great!

Recovery Words to Live By

Stay in the moment. Just let it happen
when it happens. It will happen.

Mistake #3: The Weigh-In

When we diet, we rely on the scale to measure our success. If we see any gain, even a fraction of a pound, it freaks us out. If it happens often enough, it derails our efforts. We end up thinking we're getting nowhere, and we quit trying. Why should I deprive myself if I'm going to *gain* weight, right?

Many diet gurus tell you to stay off the scale. They say you should weigh yourself no more than once a week, and some prescribe a monthly weigh-in. I threw that out the window too and approached the scale in a whole new way.

Especially in the first couple of weeks, I weighed myself often throughout the day. Morning, noon, and night, and ten times in between, I'd jump on the scale. I'll be the first to admit that was obsessive behavior, but in doing so I came to understand unequivocally that my weight fluctuates all day and night. It could go up as much as five or six pounds throughout the day but would be back to normal in the morning. That's why, for your recordable weight, it's important to weigh yourself at the same time of day. At any other time, the changing numbers you see on the scale are just normal ups and downs as your body works through its normal course of activity, day and night. I repeat, *normal* ups and downs.

Think about that for a minute. Believe me, it will reshape your attitude entirely when you start *expecting* to see the numbers rise and fall.

It used to make me a little crazy when I would weigh in at my doctor's office or at a Weight Watcher's meeting. Those appointments and meetings were typically in the late afternoon or evening, so my weight would be higher than it had been when I weighed myself that morning. I'd go into it expecting to show a loss and might instead see what would appear to be a gain. That's really frustrating and disappointing.

So it's a psychologically helpful exercise to weigh yourself often, day and night, those first few days or weeks, or however long it takes you to come to terms with the fact that your weight naturally fluctuates. You'll come to expect to see your numbers go up as the day goes on, with the full understanding that they will eventually start winding back down. Those fractions of a pound will lose all meaning. This will reduce the perceived power of the scale and let you move on without fearing it.

Another point I want to make about the scale is this: our weight—the number that appears on the scale—is just one measure of our efforts. My greater successes were in watching my body take on new shapes. You might want to measure yourself in all the key body areas so you'll have another way to see how well you are doing. I didn't do that this time, but I observed the changes as they happened and sure felt it in my clothes.

When my shoes started flipping off my feet, and when my underwear got droopy, these were tangible signs of success! I'd continue wearing baggy jeans until they were so oversized that the crotch practically hung down to my knees, partly to avoid having to buy new ones in a size I would soon outgrow and partly to hear the comments of my family. When my sister started giving me a good-natured razzing, I knew I was on the right track! It was a joyfully clear indicator of another payoff besides the scale.

I hope you have someone in your life who can do that for you. But with or without support, it's essential that you practice self-love throughout your journey.

Recovery Words to Live By

Release your inner cheerleader. Root for yourself!

Mistake #4: Seeking Validation

We don't always have someone around who will notice our losses and encourage us in continued success. Especially for those of us who have yo-yo dieted, weight loss to us is a hard-won victory, but those around us may not see it as the big deal we do, especially if they've witnessed our cycles of gains and losses many times before. And oftentimes it can take a loss of twenty pounds or more before you look much different and more than that before anyone even notices. So don't count on external reinforcement. Enjoy it when you get it, but learn to be your own advocate and champion!

Recovery Words to Live By

Talk to yourself like a friend every day throughout the day. Tell yourself all the encouraging words you want to hear.

Mistake #5: The Language

Another thing common in many diet programs that I discarded altogether was certain language associated with food. I never once said, "I can't have that," or considered any food "cheating" or "not allowed" or "off-limits." With that vocabulary, you'd naturally perceive food as the enemy. I *love* food. So that way of thinking just doesn't work for me. Also, remember, my inner junkie is a child and therefore rebellious by nature. The minute you say I "can't have" something, it's all my inner junkie is going to think about, and you can bet the farm that after much agonizing obsession on my part, we're eventually going to have it. Lots of it!

Again, psychologically, this is a massive threat to your success. When you eat the "forbidden" food, telling yourself it is "cheating" or "being bad," you feel guilty. In your psyche, you are a cheater, you are bad, and there is something wrong with you. If you do it more than once, the guilt builds up, and after repeated transgressions, you perceive yourself as a horrible failure. Why would you continue to do something that makes you feel so bad about yourself? You won't! You'll quit. And you'll likely overeat to swallow up all those negative feelings of worthlessness that cheaters, bad people, and quitters experience. Good heavens! You don't deserve that.

I don't characterize my experience as being "on a diet," because I wasn't. As my family will attest, I continued eating any foods I wanted. People might not even have known I was trying to lose weight. Internally, I was making choices and calculating risks. My choices became numbers-based, not necessarily based on the food itself. So I didn't eliminate any food entirely. I just became more selective to keep to my numbers. As a result, I ate fewer sweets and junk food. But I was free to choose. That makes all the difference.

The Food Journal—Not a Mistake at All

Another key to shifting to a meal-by-meal relationship with food is the age-old food journal. Tried and true. Most food journals are about writing down what you eat. Simple enough. This allows you to track your calories, your protein intake, your "points," or whatever element is the focus of your diet. You (or your nutritionist or diet advisor) can look back to see what foods may have impacted weight changes. During recovery, it's not just about naming the foods you eat and counting one particular characteristic. Your food journal will not only list everything you put in your mouth, it will tabulate all the nutritional information available about each morsel.

Wait—don't put this book down! If you're as much like me as I suspect, you may be balking at the idea of having to write everything down. *Please stay with me.* You most likely picked up this book because you are interested in knowing how to stop the madness of a weight problem once and for all, right? Consider every significant success in your life. Was it easy? Was the end reward handed to you at the start, or did you work hard to earn it over time? I'm guessing the hardest-won achievements were the sweetest rewards. Am I right? So why wouldn't you expect to put some effort into this critical, life-changing endeavor?

Really, how difficult is it to write down what you eat? If you'll stay with me, I'll show you how easy I have made it for you. As I said, it's very likely you will only have to do it for a few weeks. Please make that small investment in yourself.

I may not know the science of food, but there's one important thing I do know, and that is that writing down the nutritional details of the foods you eat will take the mystery out of your weight losses and gains. Information is power, and thus it will transfer the power away from the food, directly to you. That is huge. So I'll say it again, with oomph:

Keeping an honest food journal will transfer the power away from food, directly to you!

So stay with me, okay?

Okay!

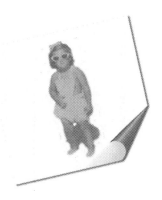

The Numbers, Meal-by-Meal

My shift from "living to eat" to "eating to live" was mostly about arming myself with information. One of the driving forces for eating more consciously was a need to lower my cholesterol. To do that, I figured I should start by knowing how much cholesterol was in my normal diet. I was blown away by what I learned. According to my research at the time, my daily intake of cholesterol should be no more than 250 milligrams a day. That sounded like a lot, until I started adding up the milligrams I was eating in my everyday foods. One egg contains about 215 mg, so two eggs for breakfast knocks it out of the park already.

Consider my Sunday omelet at the diner, made with three eggs and two slices of cheese. With one egg at 215 mg and a slice of cheddar cheese at 29 mg, my three-egg omelet had at least 703 mg! Never mind the three slices of bacon (81) and buttered toast on the side (62). We're looking at more than triple the amount of cholesterol I should be consuming, and that was just one regular meal I was eating every week. Add the home fries and the occasional pancake, and the caloric intake (1,509) should have been knocking me to the ground! That was one meal! No wonder I was a fat person with high cholesterol.

While I was now tracking cholesterol, as long as I was reading labels anyway, I figured why not also capture other nutritional information? So that's what I did, although I didn't know right away how I would use the information. I set up a spreadsheet in Excel to track calories, fat grams, saturated fat, cholesterol, sugar, protein, fiber, and sodium. (Now there are many inexpensive apps for this that will make it much less of a chore for you.) In time, these numbers helped me see food as a formula, a set of components that affect my body in ways I don't have the education to explain. They became a black-and-white image of content by gram or milligram and, in a strange way, stopped representing food. Accidentally, at some point very early on, I stopped viewing food so much as a source of pleasure and rather as a way of keeping some measure of healthy balance in my body. Imagine that!

Taking many alternative sources into account, I ultimately arrived at the following numbers as what I believed appropriate in a good daily diet for someone my age, height, weight, health, and normal activity level at the time:

Cholesterol	No more than 250 mg/day
Fiber	At least 14 g/day, 24 even better
Fat	At most 25% of daily calories from healthy fats
Sugar	Max 40 g/day of added sugar (vs. natural sugars in foods like fruit)
Sodium	Max 2,400 g/day
Calories:	1,200–1,300/day to lose weight with minimal physical effort 1,300–1,500/day to lose weight with extra physical effort

This worked for me. You need to find out what is right for you. Thereafter, you have to be diligent in monitoring your numbers meal-by-meal over the next three to four weeks. We are generally creatures of habit in our food selection, tending to eat the same foods on a weekly basis, so once you have recorded a few weeks of food intake, you should have a fairly exhaustive list of what you typically eat and the numbers associated with your normal regimen. Once you have that, the work of acquiring data is behind you. So stick with it for at least three weeks, and you should be in a good position to understand—and eventually dominate—your numbers.

So back to my Sunday breakfast example—my favorite meal to eat out. As I said, I was accustomed to a three-egg cheese omelet with bacon, two pieces of buttered toast, home fries, and occasionally a small pancake on the side. It all broke down like this:

Food	Fat/SatFat	Chol	Sodium	Carb	Fiber	Sugar	Protein	Cals
3 Eggs	15/4.5	645	210	3	0	0	21	240
2 Slices of cheese	18/12	58	348	0	0	0	14	226
3 Bacon	9/3	81	555	0	0	0	9	129
2 Toast	2/0	0	422	30	4	2	6	166
Butter	12/7	31	82	0	0	0	0	102
Home fries	9/4	23	666	35	3	3	4	230
Pancake	7/1	45	402	22	1	0	5	175
Syrup	0/0	0	80	53	0	33	0	210
Coffee/ cream	3/2	10	11	1	0	0	0	31
Total	**75/33.5**	**893**	**2,776**	**144**	**8**	**38**	**59**	**1,509**

In one meal, I took in a full day's calories and far exceeded fat, cholesterol, and sodium allotments for an entire day. Wow! If I was to reduce my cholesterol, this would have to stop. And if I wanted to lose weight, I had to ask myself, "What can I do to change this?" The answer was elementary, nothing new, just the simple facts we already know to be true:

To lower my cholesterol, I needed to make different selections, exchanging high-number foods for lower-number foods whenever possible. So if I still wanted an omelet, I'd request Egg Beaters or have it made with egg whites only; I would load it with veggies and *one* slice of cheese and could hardly tell the difference.

To lose weight, I had to manage my portion sizes in relation to how many calories I was expending. I still eat eggs, but one instead of three. If I want a real fried egg, I eat a real fried egg. And yes, I still eat cheese, but a few slices per week instead of per meal. I also still eat toast, generally choosing higher fiber bread and sometimes using jelly instead of butter. I still eat home fries too but might eat only a half portion. And if I'm in the mood for a pancake, I might substitute it for the toast and/or potatoes.

Those small changes make a massive difference:

Food	Fat/SatFat	Chol	Sodium	Carb	Fiber	Sugar	Protein	Cals
1 Egg	5/1.5	215	70	1	0	0	7	80
2 Toast	2/0	0	140	26	6	4	6	166
Jelly	12/7	0	0	13	0	12	0	50
Home fries	4.5/2	11.5	333	17.5	1.5	1.5	3	115
Coffee/cream	3/2	10	11	1	0	0	0	31
Total	**26.5/12.5**	**236.5**	**554**	**58.5**	**7.5**	**17.5**	**16**	**442**

The menu is all up to me, and it's ever changeable. It's all about keeping to my daily numbers. I still drink coffee with cream. For some reason, I feel more satiated when I finish a meal that way. I don't have bacon often, but that's just a choice I make. I never tell myself I can't have it. I just acknowledge that a serving of three slices has 81 grams of cholesterol, 3 grams of saturated fat, and 129 calories, and it sometimes loses its appeal. Funny how that happens.

So as you can see, I still eat a satisfying breakfast, but it's one meal in a meal-by-meal approach. I just do my best to balance my numbers by the end of the day. If I overdo any given meal, I have the next meal to offset it. If I want to throw caution to the wind, that's my choice, though it's a choice I rarely ever make anymore. Whatever I do, the next meal is my opportunity to manage my numbers successfully. That's the way it works, meal-by-meal.

You might think that the ability to redeem yourself at the next meal would give you license to approach a meal carelessly. Well, honestly, in a way it does. But I hope you'll find yourself so engrossed in making the numbers work that you won't want that to happen. And you'll be enjoying weight-loss successes on a regular basis that will keep you motivated to continue a numbers-based approach. The good news is that if you do choose to overdo, you can leave that meal behind and focus on the next one to do what's best for you. Don't berate yourself for the occasional misstep. Accept it and move on.

If there's one commitment you must make to your recovery—or any weight-loss program—it is that you must be absolutely honest with yourself about what you eat. It won't do you any good to pretend a small bite of something never happened. As hard as I've tried to make it so, ignoring little morsels does not make them magically disappear. There are numbers (and consequences) associated with every bite, big or small. If you don't account for them, your efforts will be a lie and will do you no good whatsoever.

Until you have a perfect understanding of your food habits, formulated over several weeks, everything—and I mean everything—must be taken into account: the milk you splash on your cereal, the oil you drizzle in the pan before cooking, the handful of nuts you nibble as you're watching TV. Everything. Bite by bite.

♥

At the time I mastered eating meal-by-meal, I had been involuntarily unemployed for several months. About three months in, I was talking to a cousin about unemployment and potentially being forced by economics to sell my home. I remarked on how surprising it was that I, as an emotional eater, was able to lose weight so successfully at a time when I was feeling so sad, frightened, and helpless. To my own amazement, I heard myself utter these words: "I feel like what I put in my mouth is the only thing I can control right now."

OMG! Somebody get Oprah on the phone! Talk about your aha moments.

You think you can't control the food you eat, but it's really one of the few things in life you *can* control. You can't control the traffic that sets off your stress; you can't control the spouse who brings unhealthy foods into the house; you can't control the illness that sends a loved one to the hospital; you can't control the colleague who undermines you at work; you can't control anything other than yourself.

Meal-by-meal, pound-by-pound, you will seize that control.

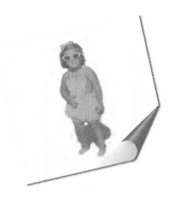

Step-by-Step:
THE E WORD

Whatever you do, don't tell me I have to exercise. It might get ugly! If you're reading this, chances are that very word grates on your nerves too. I threw that out the window with the others.

Listen, if you love to work out at the gym, I'm really happy for you and encourage you to continue to do so. Or maybe you like to play a sport, ride a bike, or get a workout in some other fun way. That's great! When I'm motivated, which is admittedly infrequent, I like to tap dance, and for a while I was an avid swimmer. But many, many people who are overweight don't engage that way. Even calling it a "workout" sets some of us up to view it negatively.

We do have to burn calories to shed or minimize fat and lose weight. There's just no way around it. We have to put in some physical effort. For my recovery, I turned to a simple, age-old solution: I walk.

I started from nothing. The only movement my body knew at night was getting from the refrigerator to the couch and the couch to the bed. I'm not kidding. I was utterly immobile. My breathing would get labored from just going up the stairs to do my laundry. And I must confess the worst, most incredibly embarrassing effect: because of my weight, I often snorted loudly, especially when I laughed. My big belly obstructed my breathing, reducing air intake, causing me to force air through my nose … and snort. Truly mortifying.

So if you are at zero, I wholeheartedly empathize with your probable fear of movement. When you're completely inactive and out of shape, like I was, it's scary to think of getting physical. It is likely that you may also believe you are too far gone to turn things around. Not so. I promise.

For those of you who are inactive and want to get started on your own recovery, I challenge you to get up and walk. In fact, put this book down for a few minutes, dress for the weather, go outside, and take a walk. Walk whatever small distance is comfortable—walking no longer than ten minutes round-trip. If you get winded, stop, rest, and slowly walk home. If walking to your mailbox is the farthest you can go without stress, so be it. Make the mailbox first base. For now, that's all there is to it.

Later, when you are comfortable walking to the mailbox—or wherever your first steps took you—you will move a little farther. You'll set your sights on a tree, a telephone pole, a crossroad, anything that will extend your walk a little bit farther each day.

If you have a pedometer, it's kind of fun to track your distance. Believe it or not, you're likely to build up to walking close to two miles a day. But don't obsess over distance. With food you go meal-by-meal, with weight you go pound-by-pound, and with movement you simply go step-by-step. Each time you are able to walk a few more steps, set a goal to walk a few more than that. And when you reach that goal, add a few more steps.

♥

My daily walk is convenient and simple. That's what you should aim for, since you'll stay committed if it isn't an ordeal. If your home location is not suitable for walking, you might have to go elsewhere, like a mall or a park, but if at all possible, walk your own extended neighborhood. Walking the blocks around my home has ensured that my walk is expedient and enjoyable. My pace and distance are set by my mood, health, weather, and personal choice on any given day. Don't pressure yourself whatsoever.

Over time, I have tracked four distinctly different routes for myself, and I suggest you do the same. This ensures that if the weather is unpleasant or you don't want to make the time or your walking campaign feels routine or you have a dozen other real or imagined excuses, you will have options. You can choose which route you're able and willing to walk.

The Core Route—First Base:

This is what you will build up to during your first day(s) or week(s) of walking. It should be a short, pleasant, ten-minute walk. The distance is entirely up to you and your body, but once it's established, promise yourself you will walk nothing less than your core route each and every day. My core route is just under half a mile. If I am pressed for time or don't feel like walking (which rarely happens these days), I walk the core only and call it a successful day.

The Basic Route—Second Base:

This will add another ten minutes and be at least double the distance of your core. My basic route adds four large, residential blocks and is a little over a mile. It has a small incline that winded me at first. It took awhile to build up to it, but now it is effortless. That's the beauty of walking. The more you do, the more your body is able to do. The more you are able to do, the more you will want to do.

The Extended Route—Third Base:

My extended route adds another ten minutes and a small hill.

The Full Route—Home Run:

This is the full monty! My full route takes about forty minutes and is just under two miles. That's just slightly longer, and much more rewarding, than the time spent watching one sitcom or reality show rerun. (Yes, I *know* you!) It includes a large hill that took me weeks to tackle without trepidation and months to build the stamina needed to conquer it without huffing and puffing. You won't believe how fabulous it will feel to become that kind of conqueror. Go forth and conquer!

I have found these months later that on the few occasions when I'm not enthused about walking, I leave the house intending to do only the core. I promised myself I'd do at least that every day. It's just ten quick minutes. Now that it's habitual, once I get started, my internal dialogue goes something like this:

"I'm proud of you for doing the core when you really don't feel like it. Great job!"

"Yeah, I'm very proud of myself."

"What number do you want to see next on the scale?"

"Well, since I weighed 173 this morning, I want to see 172."

"That would be great! You know, to see 172 without cutting back on calories, you need to walk more than your core route."

"Yeah, I know. Well, now that I'm out, I might as well do a little more and walk a bigger route."

"Excellent! You're doing an amazing job."

When I think that way, I tend to do the *full* route and am always so proud and happy with myself for showing that commitment. I know there will be a payoff that is worth those extra steps. A big part of the payoff is the stimulation of those dopamine-producing neurons, as well as the release of endorphins that essentially create a natural high—a massive, lasting sense of satisfaction that you genuinely want to repeat. I've essentially traded food addiction for an addiction to walking. It's my saving grace.

Physically, I've gone from this: to this: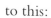

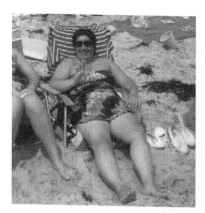 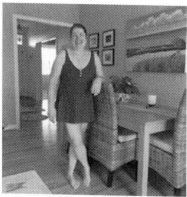

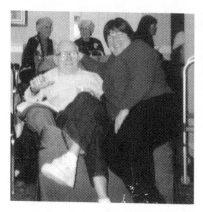 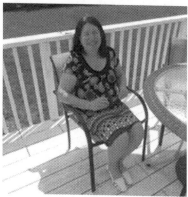

And the journey continues …

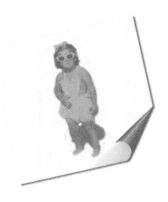

Addiction

Food addiction is a lifelong affliction. It's not something that just goes away. Even if you were to wake up skinny tomorrow, the temptation to make poor choices and overeat will always exist. You know it, and I know it. Every roller-coaster dieter and food junkie knows it. It's the nature of the beast.

Consider the alcoholic. Once someone is in the throes of this disease, she will always and forever be an alcoholic. She may stop drinking, God willing, but a period of sobriety does not end her acutely perilous relationship with alcohol. At Alcoholics Anonymous, sobriety is celebrated one day at a time ... for life. One hopes that it becomes less and less monstrous the longer one stays sober, but the monster has not been killed, merely quieted. If you are a food junkie, you will celebrate healthy food choices meal-by-meal, standing up to your monster one meal at a time.

Knowing your struggle as I do, I want so badly for you to have the healthy life I am finally enjoying. If you don't accept your addiction for the reckoning force that it is, you could so easily fall off the wagon and undo the good, clean living that recovery can help you enjoy. Please don't let the mechanics stop you from finally realizing your best self.

AFTER

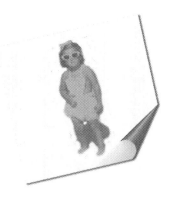

The Holy Grail

I couldn't fully explain my recovery without addressing those elements of food and movement, the walking mechanics of time and distance, and the mathematical equation of calories in and calories out. However, none of that comes remotely close to conveying the next, most significant, discovery. Looking back at all my other attempts to sustain weight loss, food and movement are shockingly meaningless without the most critical component: spiritual healing.

My mother was a devout Catholic. I admired her profound love of God and devotion to her faith. These are priceless gifts that she passed on to me, and I am eternally grateful.

"What's to be, will be" was a mantra she reiterated often throughout my life. She firmly believed everything happened for a reason, governed by God's plan for each of us, and we saw that realized many times over. In line with that belief, I have a small, painted tile on my bureau that reads: "Trust God. You are exactly where you are meant to be."

Just before my recovery began, I bottomed out again. I was feeling exhausted and beaten down by years of living a workaday life that did not feed my spirit. My job was all-consuming, a chronic source of discontent. My moral compass was overpowered and trampled by greed, aggression, politics, and ethical conflict. Simultaneously, tragedy and loss had piled up over the years. In succession, I suffered a devastating house fire, my car was totaled in a winter storm, my mother had a debilitating stroke, my one and only child moved to the West Coast, my father died, I was fired from my job, my cat was hit and killed by a car, my mother died, my sister got cancer, I lost another job in a corporate acquisition, and my cottage near the shore was taken by the bank.

Heartbreak piled up relentlessly, stacked like massive, concrete dominoes falling with deafening force, one against the other. I hadn't recovered from one before the next hit the ground. I was eating my way into oblivion.

When all was said and done, I fell hard and deep into despair. Utterly broken down, I looked at that pretty little tile one day and considered hurling it against the wall. I tearfully challenged all that I'd believed. This couldn't possibly be where I was meant to be! I raged, "God, this is your genius plan for me?"

♥

Without faith, there is no hope. My life imploded, dissolved into a puddle of muck and mire, to where I could barely lift my feet to move ahead. I could hardly see my way out of bed for weeks.

Enter Sister Joan Reilly. Sister Joan was a nun who had served at my church. I saw her every Sunday and every holiday for many, many years, but the only time we had ever talked was when she helped arrange the Mass for my mother's funeral years earlier, after which I stopped going to church. Little did I know at the time, we were kindred spirits meant to be reunited.

With concern for my deepening depression, and knowing my funds were dwindling, my sister sought a referral for me from a family friend to a counseling service called Conversations Inc. at the Sisters of Saint Joseph convent. Reluctantly, I made an appointment. When I recognized Sister Joan ambling down the corridor to greet me, I was overcome by a knowing rush of comfort. God had led me there.

Sister Joan has a way of moving me that contributed immensely to my recovery. For the next eighteen months, she walked me through the darkness, talked me through the shadows, and danced with me when I returned to the light. I threw my heartaches into space; she caught them with a knowing grace. And thus the puzzle was complete.

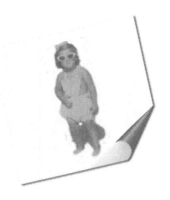

The Epiphany

Early on in my recovery, I realized that the time I spent walking had ceased to be just about burning calories. It had become cherished time spent healing the wounds of my inner junkie—that sweet, precious child hiding in closets and sneaking about to feed her loneliness and pain. In my reflections on the past, I gave witness to her desperation and aloneness over the years and wished I could go back in time to scoop her up in my arms and hold her tight. For the first time in my life, I felt a resolute compassion for myself, and I was compelled to reclaim and nurture the child within. I began to model Sister Joan's loving, affirming ways whenever I encountered my inner junkie. I made it my mission to love her, guide her, reassure her, and protect her, from here forward. That resolve has changed me forever.

I use my walking time to nourish myself. I replace shaming, disapproving messages of the past with words of acceptance and encouragement. I remind myself that I am a child of God, the most divine Holy Spirit, who made me and loves me exactly as I am. I have helped my inner junkie to see that we are eternally in God's care, never alone. We talk with God as we walk, each honoring the other with abiding love. This knowledge has created contentment beyond words as I enjoy a newfound sense of harmony and immense gratitude.

I know now that the primary object I've been seeking all these years is not a new body size or weight or even power over food. The principal foundation of the quest was peace for my soul. Without that, I could not succeed at genuine, lasting restoration. It is liberating. It is joyful. A miraculous reawakening! Think Dorothy Gale, waking up back home in Kansas, her beloved Toto safe in her arms, her adoring family at her bedside. Think Indiana Jones, gazing upon the Holy Grail after tumultuous years of searching and believing.

I liken my journey to the epiphany, as it is profoundly, exquisitely described in this poem by Joyce Rupp[*]:

[*]   Excerpted from: Rupp, Joyce. *Out of the Ordinary*. Notre Dame, IN: Ave Maria Press, 2011. Used with permission of the publisher.

Epiphany
(Matthew 2:1–12)

they listened deep inside,
far into the darkness
where even a tiny bit of light
seemed like sunburst in the heart.

they pondered the silent music
that echoed in their prayer:
"Go. Search. Look. Follow. Find."

a journey without precedent,
adventure wrought with risk,
a time of travel filled with faith.

they went lovingly, eagerly,
into the night of their lives,
trusting they would find the way.

they paused to inquire, to study,
they went on in faith, patiently,
following with the hearts' eye.

and "the sight of the star
filled them with delight."

a journey not in vain,
a patient search rewarded,

their steady courage in the unknown
led them to their heart's delight.

they found the long-sought One,
waiting to be found,
longing to be discovered,
as they traveled the far stretches
of their long and hidden night.

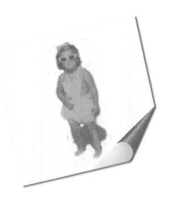

Habit Breakers

If you're eating meal-by-meal and walking step-by-step with God, you'll see miraculous changes in your life. But you may still find yourself occasionally eating for comfort. Not to worry! It's temporary. In time, with a new consciousness, with practice and dedication, you'll find yourself doing less and less of it.

Honestly, food has not been my go-to partner in over a year, despite going through some tough emotional battles. I never imagined this to be possible. I've kicked the habit by employing one or more of the following practices whenever the potential for emotional eating looms:

Acknowledge any mindless or out-of-control eating.

By paying close attention to your habits over the next few weeks, you'll become much more mindful of what you put in your mouth. Awareness is the first big step in breaking the habit.

Feel your feelings.

You are entitled to your feelings. They are a big part of what makes you human. If something makes you mad, feel mad! If you are sad, feel sad. Whatever you're feeling, you have a right to it. Give yourself permission to feel whatever you feel. It's okay. Recognize that it's a temporary state.

Talk to a friend.

If you have a friend who listens well, talk it out. Articulate the circumstances, the who/what/when/where/why—every relevant detail. Express how it made you feel. Sometimes all we need is to be heard.

Talk to yourself.

Let your internal dialogue reflect the tender, loving care you deserve. Whatever emotion has you off-balance, ask yourself what you would do for or say to a friend or loved one feeling that way and then do or tell yourself exactly that. Let your inner voice become your best friend.

Pray.

Turn to God. Ask for support and guidance. Pray that you will be strong enough to get through the emotions of the moment without turning to food. Earnest prayer is very soothing and comforting. And the act of praying will put some time, distance, and reflection between you and food. By the time your meditation is over, you will be much less agitated, more reasonable, and far less inclined to stuff your face with food.

Walk.

Go where food is not available. Stew if you have to—get it out. Shake it off or cry it out with a full route's walk. Very soon, you'll feel differently about things.

Whenever you can, combine prayer and walking. It's a healing practice that offers a multitude of rewards.

Count your blessings.

Observe and ponder all the good things in your life. It is rich with blessings if you'll only take the time to appreciate them. Develop an attitude of gratitude. Carry thanksgiving in your heart, and include thankfulness in your communications with God. Doing this on a regular basis will change everything.

♥

Of course, we need to be realistic and accept the fact that we might very well get too swept up in something emotional to talk or pray or walk. You may end up feeding the turmoil. When that happens, let it be, friend. Just let it be. When your head is clear again, simply and privately concede that your emotions temporarily took control. Forgive yourself and recognize that the world did not come to an end. Calculate the intake as part of your day, and move on. If the numbers are outrageous, don't agonize over them. Put them behind you, and just move on.

Emotional eating is a habit that takes lots of practice and effort to break. If you're like me, it's been your modus operandi for years. Don't expect it to vanish into thin air just because you want it to. And remember, you are retraining your brain—no small task. As I said, with a new consciousness, with practice and perseverance, you'll find it happening much less often. It takes time to break a habit, especially one that has been a longstanding way of life.

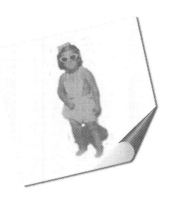

Final Words

I still have miles to go on this journey, but the small accomplishments along the way are proving not to be small at all. They are building, one on the other, and I'm achieving repeated successes and deep personal satisfaction as I go.

I hope you find my experience helpful in creating your own path to recovery. May it release your authentic, unencumbered self and deliver you to your dream destination.

♥

Three weeks ago, I celebrated the completion of the first draft of this book with a Buster Bar ice cream treat from Dairy Queen. I ate it publicly, right there at the DQ picnic tables, with kids and adults all around me. I savored every lick and mouthful, without embarrassment, shame, guilt, or remorse. I chalked up the 460 calories and walked my full route twice that day. It was worth every step. With the grace of God, I have not longed for anything else extravagant in the weeks since. It was very, very delicious and satisfying … lip-smacking good.